C000015856

A Bite-Sized Lifestyle Book

Cancer –
Living Behind Enemy Lines
Without a Map

Bill Heine

Published by Bite-Sized Books Ltd 2018

**Registered in the UK. Company Registration No: 9395379
ISBN: 9781718172838**

Bite-Sized Books Ltd Cleeve Croft, Cleeve Road, Goring RG8 9BJ UK
information@bite-sizedbooks.com

With grateful acknowledgment to the
Oxford Mail
for permission to republish these
articles.

Contents

Introduction

Cancer is a foreign country; and yes, they do things differently there.

They feed you poison and call it hope. They keep you in the dark so others can see your problem more clearly. They don't tell you to prepare for life or death.

I live in this foreign country. This is the story of how I got there and what it's doing to me.

Maybe it's a funny book.

Chapter 1

Where Do We Go from Here?

10th November 2017

This will be a short book; I have terminal cancer.

Spoiler alert! I'm still alive.

The story is based on columns I wrote for the Oxford Mail and unfolds exactly as it did for me.

None of us knows how we will react if we get the disease that will kill 2 out of 3 of us, but I found out...accidentally.

During a blood test at the Churchill Hospital when I was wired to a machine and couldn't escape, one of the nurses who didn't expect to see me, entered the huge treatment hall, spotted me and came straight up. I recognized her as part of a team organized to monitor my symptoms.

She was flushed and on a bit of a high. "I've just this moment come from a team meeting discussing you," she announced with the excitement of a presenter at the Academy Awards to proclaim *and the winner is*. "You've got leukaemia and if ever there is a good time to have leukaemia, this is it!!

"A slew of new drugs to treat it is coming down the pipeline and there are options to take part in trials with experimental, state of the art drugs."

She was totally positive and lifted my spirits. For a while I did believe I had won something.

Two days later my partner of thirty odd years, Jane, and I met the consultant. He didn't know the nurse had tipped us off. We sat in his office like two little minnows on a hook as be came straight to the point.

"I'm sorry to have to tell you but you have acute myeloid leukaemia known in the medical profession as AML."

He explained how the disease worked and asked the killer question: "Do you want to talk about your length of life?"

I now know well into the treatment regime that a lot of patients prefer to pass on that one.

Somewhere deep inside most of us is a hopeful, but fanciful idea of how long we can expect to live. Where we pluck these numbers from is anyone's guess but I, perhaps foolheartedly, thought I would last between ten to fifteen years with the leukaemia, but Jane and I hadn't discussed nor thought about this obvious question.

How do you feel when your cancer consultant tells you the average life expectancy is twelve to eighteen months? Well, the years fly away and the film of your life that unfolds in your head blows up.

Suddenly everything that was warm and connected and clear becomes cold, lonely and confusing.

I didn't know where to go with this news, but neither did Jane. She was not just pale, but deathly white.

I headed to the nearest escape hatch. "You said there were some treatments. How much more time will that give me?"

He answered in a dead-pan manner and when the resonance of his voice faded away, it left a scum, "The treatment benefit is factored into the mortality rate, so nothing changes."

He went on to give me some life-style advice. It was like trying to do a Tango with Dr. No and every time you got anywhere he would stop the music and nail your foot to the floor.

His opening gambit was about cleanliness: "You know you have no immune system to speak of. So you're an easy target for any bug or germ you've heard of and many you have not.

"If you've ever wanted to know about fantastic micro-beasts and where to find them, look around. You are the best bit of bait to attract them."

Jane interrupted, "We live in a converted tithe barn and at this time of year the field mice start moving inside for the winter. We're both busy. Bill does interviews and I run a pottery, so every once in a while our barn resembles a pig sty."

After discovering this chink in our anti-cancer armour, he started to probe for other weaknesses: "How much alcohol do you drink"?

I told him that most people lied to their doctor about alcohol consumption, after all Oxford is a city that is partly fuelled by wine, sherry, beer, brandy and port. But I told him the truth and his reply was generous, "That's not too bad. That's all right."

Then I decided to get some answers from him. "What if I smoked? Would you say that was all right?" This tends to be a hard question for any medical person because they have to weigh up the harm against the pleasure in the particular case.

"I know it's difficult if you are addicted," started the consultant, squirming and wriggling. "I won't say *stop* because if this helps you deal with cancer it may be a good thing. However if you pull through the cancer treatment it would be hard to see you die of a stroke from smoking. But since you have such little time left..."

Jane couldn't bear it any longer. "Doctor, he doesn't smoke!"

That's true but I needed to ask my consultant whether or not he really was serious about the twelve to eighteen months of life left. I wanted to test the edges of that time limit to find out if there was any hope somewhere; and he went against his convictions as a medical professional and said, "Keep smoking if you want and enjoy it. Time is limited."

By taking the smoking question in a balanced way instead of saying *just give up the habit*, he gave me no choice. I had to believe him. This was a game-changer. There was no way out of this one – except in a coffin.

We heard no talk of the exciting new wonder drugs, no mention of world class research trials of experimental drugs carried out at Oxford University Hospitals. There was only Dr. No putting his foot firmly down on my *hope pipe*.

Jane and I left in silence and decided to have lunch at my favourite deli in Thame – *What's Cooking?*. We didn't say anything till we sat down to share a bowl of their lettuce, pea and Thai satay soup.

I held her hand and said, "Well, this is one of those life-changing events."

"Yes," she said quietly and quickly. "So is death."

We laughed a little and had a long, delicious lunch.

Chapter 2

Dr Yes

17th November 2017

The man who called us back to his office the following week had changed his spots to read *Dr Yes*. He asked casually if I would be interested in going on a drug trial to help discover a new treatment for my kind of leukaemia. I would be part of an experiment with 110 people.

Humph -- I thought – 110 people in Oxfordshire sounds like a small and maybe insignificant trial.

My hopes were still sliding down a hole when Dr Yes explained it was a world-wide trial and the 110 people came from across the globe. Only two others were from Oxfordshire.

There were lots of barriers stopping anyone from joining the trial. First we had to confirm the lists were still open and they were prepared to take new participants. Next I needed to pass the physical entry tests like heart, liver and lung condition. Third I must meet the drug company criteria for this specific illness.

Finally, even if I managed to hop through all these hoops, I may not get the new, exciting drug treatment because only half of the people accepted for the trial get it. There is no mystery. All participants know who is on the experimental drug and who is not.

During one cliff hanger of a week I took all the tests and found out I passed them all. Eventually official looking emails came from Switzerland and the United States confirming that I was to get the new drug. The other two participants in the Oxfordshire area, who had been on the trial for six months, did not get the new drug.

Just 23 hours later the Trials Nurse received notification that the particular window of opportunity offered by this trial drug had been slammed shut.

I must have been one of the last of *the lucky gang*. I felt like Gary Cooper in *High Noon*, the gun slinging sheriff in a duel to the death, where the other guy pulled the trigger first but the bullet ricocheted off the badge on my chest and saved my life, maybe. Up yours, death... At least for the time being. But I knew this duel was far from over.

What exactly was I getting with this *trial*? I am getting two drugs for one week and then nothing for three weeks. This treatment process is repeated for four months.

The two drugs include the leading licensed drug currently fighting many forms of leukaemia. This kind of drug had not improved much in the last thirty years This leading drug is not specifically targeted at leukaemia but hits every cell in the body and poisons them. But some leukaemia patients respond positively to this treatment.

I asked my consultant if this sounded like a medieval punishment that people would not even administer to Jesus Christ. He remained silent.

This *top of the range drug* did not appear to be an answer to the disease. Hence the search and trial for a new drug that would specifically target the cancer cells, put a protein marker on the outside of those cancer cells so the usual drug of the past thirty years would be attracted to zap the cancer cells.

This sounds logical and a major advance to kill the cancer cells but when I look at my quiet, calm, deceptively tranquil arms and hands I know, in the veins I can see just beneath the skin, a major battle of my survival is playing out and a kind of war is going on.

A trial is a gamble. We don't know how this will turn out. It may be a miracle treatment for many cancers or it may fizzle out as a major hope lost.

The physical results probably won't be in evidence for some time, but the economic effects are already clear. The new drug costs around £85,000 per year per patient. Currently the drug companies absorb this cost, but if the drug works and is licensed in the UK, will the NHS be allowed to purchase it by the financial and clinical watchdog agency – NICE – the National Institute for Clinical Excellence? In other words will the drug be worth the cost?

One of the reasons to write this column is that we usually hear very little about the *trial* process of a new drug. We hear only a brief sentence or two to summarize the results published in medical journals. But we don't hear the real, rollercoaster ride taken by patients on the trials. Too often there is a disconnect between the triumphant results and the reality of the foot soldiers in the front line.

And what about my cancer consultant, Dr No? The Trial Nurse told me that when she confirmed to him I was selected for the trial, he punched the air and said "Yes! Yes! Yes!"

Chapter 3

Drawing Blood

24th November 2017

I woke up with a sense of heavenly bliss and relief that the first two cycles of my cancer treatment were over. All I had to do today was have a blood test at 10.00 in the morning

How difficult can that be? I weighted up my options. This should take ten minutes to draw the nine vials of blood and an extra one for the miracle machine at the Churchill Hospital that can give you a detailed profile of yourself in 5 minutes to alert staff if you need a blood transfusion tomorrow, which they had already booked, just in case.

All very efficient!

That's the drill—15 minutes in and out, so I could park my car in the *drop off and run*, short stay, 20 minute bay just outside the entrance to my treatment centre.

But I had a premonition and didn't.

Twenty minutes turned into two hours.

I'm petrified of needles. When the trainee nurse put the canula in my left arm I looked away at the far end of the treatment hall to study the black, green and red headdress worn by the white North Oxford woman who gave off signals saying *I'm going to beat this*

The trainee nurse said I had *great veins*. That chat-up line conjured an image of Dracula's daughter, as she tightened the tourniquet and spent the next 45 minutes poking around trying to coax a few drops of blood from my veins.

Little things mean a lot -- the beads of sweat on her face, the flush of red blotches on her neck and, after half an hour, the unmistakable trembling of her thumb and forefinger.

She abandoned the left arm half an hour later and shifted the onslaught to my right which already had so many needle marks it looked like the arm of a heroin addict.

She found another big vein and delved in with the help of a support nurse. Forty five minutes later they were in worse shape than I was, and I wanted to give them some encouragement. So instead of asking *have you ever had this much trouble with anyone else?* I asked if they had *helped any other patient who was as difficult as I was*. Both nurses were well past the state where irony made any difference and unselfconsciously shook their heads vigorously. They didn't look up or smile and just said, "No."

Shortly they gave up and asked the head nurse to draw my blood, which she did in two minutes. But this vein catcher had an unexpected twist in her sobriety.

I discovered this when I enquired of the Head Nurse if she had had any unpleasant childhood memory of needles, like I had when my whole school was getting vaccinated against polio and the boy in front of me in the queue turned brilliant green-white and collapsed completely during the experience. He hit the gym floor with a thud that resonated around the room.

I had a front row seat and I could see exactly what happened. When the nurse pulled the syringe out of this fourteen year old boy's upper arm, the needle was bent at a 45% angle. With the enthusiasm, abandonment and showmanship of a novice cricket bowler, the American nurse had hit the bone. I was supposed to be next, but they weren't able to catch me.

Fortunately I had this conversation after the Head Nurse had drawn my blood This story obviously hit a nerve with her. She froze and kept saying *OMG…OMG…OMG*, and then her story came tumbling out. "I was 7 years old when my school also had a mass vaccination programme. I too ran away but the nurse snagged me by the arm and dragged me back. I'll never forget it. I guess I was traumatised."

That's when I discovered the head nurse was not only a devout Catholic who could not bring herself to say the word *God* in public and in anger, hence the *OMG…OMG*. She was fiendishly afraid of needles herself, and she also had a huge shopping list of other items fraught with fear.

In the run-up to Halloween the top prize on her list went to ghosts and haunted houses. I know a few Oxfordshire villages where locals tell stories of the supernatural, but this woman lived through the tales and bought into them. Yes, ghosts were real and houses were haunted.

She would never wear anything red to a funeral because that would show joy and happiness at the death. And you must not let your tears fall on the casket because that would unleash evil spirits.

What gives the carer the courage to dig deep into these very private areas? The relationship between two people in this intimate act of caring, during this dance macabre, when life unfolds and finishes, is unexpected, quirky and strangely direct.

Great! If you're going to go to hell in a handcart, it's probably better to have someone at the helm who not only shares your fears and phobias but who has travelled this bumpy road before and knows some of the potholes.

And I'll have a few things to say about pot in the future….

Chapter 4

Alternative Treatments – and Cannabis

1st December 2017

Deadlines, like being told you have between 12 and 18 months to live, mean you have nothing to lose, so why not try alternative treatments?

Can cannabis help control cancer?

That is the question posed to me by an ardent but anonymous fan who read these columns.

My number one fan has sent several medical articles arguing that pot can kill leukaemia cells.

Since cannabis is an illegal drug it is difficult to carry out experiments with it and get hard medical evidence.

I have interviewed one Oxfordshire woman who swears it has helped her during chemotherapy, especially with the nausea that is provoked by the treatment.

She says cannabis helps her to walk, talk and taste food.

Anecdotal evidence like this may not be convincing because anyone can make up a cannabis story.

There are some very powerful people in the medical profession who have studied the effects of cannabis and argue that it should be legal for medicinal purposes.

Among these people is David Knott, formerly the Chief Scientific Adviser to the Government.

Some would go further and argue that cannabis should be legalised for recreational use, or harm reduction.

This would stop the drugs money going to criminals who run drug cartels and it would provide safer drugs because cannabis could be tested and approved so that too pure or adulterated drugs, would not be available on the street.

But let's stick with cannabis for medicinal use.

There is a Catch 22 situation here. It can't be tested because it is illegal but it may be helpful, so what would you do if an anonymous fan offered to bake you two dozen hash brownies, so you wouldn't have to smoke it, just lazily munch some of the weed?

That's what my number one fan is offering. This person has thought it out. They must remain anonymous and we can have no direct contact.

So he or she will drop off the cannabis in a tin at a secret location behind a stone in the porch of a Church of England church.

I checked out the views on this with my cancer consultant and the consultant suggested that taking cannabis, as far as he knows, will nor retard or interfere with the current drugs I am taking.

Now before avid parishioners in Oxford start to get out their metal detectors and begin to comb around churchyards inch by inch please note I have rejected the offer of a regular supply of cannabis brownies, at least for the time being.

But this does bring up a deeper drugs story in my fight against leukaemia.

Several months ago, before I had a diagnosis I had a scratchy skin condition that doctors later suggested was probably related to my cancer.

My GP prescribed a regular supply of creams to combat the condition.

These drugs have all been tested and licensed by the Government and come with a list of side effects.

One of the creams, which is widely used for a variety of skin problems, has a very short list of side effects and does not flag up any dangerous associations.

I have been slapping it on all over my body for a year because the directions say *apply two to four times daily* and use as a soap substitute.

However, there are one or two problems with this cream. If you use it regularly layers and deposits of it can build up on the skin.

If you don't take a shower for two or three days this can result in a big residue.

Also, if you put it on before dressing or going to bed, your clothes and bedclothes could retain some of the cream and after a while become soaked in it.

This is when the little problem with this medically tested and licensed drug came to light, a very big light.

The problem with the cream I was using is that some of the paraffin ingredients could ignite if a flame or very hot object came in contact with it.

One man with a skin condition used it just before he went outside to light a cigarette.

He went up in flames like a torch, and with over 80 per cent burns to his body he died.

In recent years five people have died as a result of burns after using the cream.

This is a tale of two medicines.

One is cannabis, that could in certain circumstances be helpful to the human body, and which is illegal and therefore cannot be used in experiments to prove whether or not it is beneficial in treating cancer.

The second drug is legal and has had all the tests enabling me to use it with my cancer but it burned five people alive.

It is not easy being a patient because all drugs have side effects.

But if patients are to be denied the use of cannabis the regulators have some hard questions to answer about the balance of harm and help.

Maybe that's why I have not entirely ruled out finding a tin of cannabis brownies in some pot of gold hidden in a church porch.

Chapter 5

Hospital at Home

8th December 2017

Being diagnosed with leukaemia and given 12 to 18 months to live is a tight timeline to fight not only cancer but the added infections that pop up along the way. So my consultant team at the hospital asked a group of nurses and paramedics to treat me in my own bed for a week to give me extended intravenous drip treatments after my day on the wards.

The *Hospital at Home* team used an ironing board to prepare the needles and medications while I created a makeshift pallet for myself. Then we scoured the ceiling beams to find a hook to hang a bag of antibiotics.

A hand-carved white elephant wooden marionette I brought back from Bangkok 25 years ago did the trick. We shook off the dust and hoisted the bag to allow the drip-feed tube to fall into my lap and then clamped it into a semi-permanent tube I've been living with, stretching from my elbow to just above my heart.

It was all Heath Robinson and a bit *over the top* but it worked because of the intimate, caring relationship between nurse and patient.

In the 45 minutes when the antibiotics dripped into my body the carers started another drip feed operation. They sat down next to me and got out their questionnaires to pull out of me a verbal picture of my health

It's hard to refuse this especially since the nurses have gone to so much trouble. Why not co-operate with them on their homework?

I know they mean well and want to get a rounded picture of the patient, but why do these pointed questions leave a slightly sinister atmosphere hanging around afterwards? The nurses always smile when they go through this litany.

"Can you get out of bed by yourself with no assistance?" Well, yes, you've just seen me do close to a hand stand to get into this position on the mattress.

"Is your skin still moist and can you walk up the stairs without becoming dizzy or breathless and can you use a toilet unaided?"

These questions leave me with some picture they expect me to walk into in the future -- a desiccated man with sunken cheeks emphasizing the hollow rings of my eyes, collapsed on the staircase and clutching the banister while trying to retrieve a roll of toilet paper from the upstairs airing cupboard.

The next time anyone in a white or blue hospital coat with soft, doe-like, sensitive eyes puts a hand out to touch me on the arm or shoulder and asks in a very concerned voice, after taking a deep sigh – *How are you? How are you feeling?* – I may scream. At the very least I will think of joining a gym. That way I could give them the amount of weight I'm bench pressing each day this week so they could compare that figure with the tally for last week and make up their own minds about their key question *How are you feeling?*

The one thin thread that keeps me vaguely interested in these questions is that at least they have the merit of being clear.

Then on the last day of my treatment the medical team waived that advantage *good bye.*

A nurse with no great interest in her final question asked me: "Are you a message in a bottle?" and she didn't even blink when I asked her to repeat it.

She caught me off guard. "Maybe, but what exactly do you mean?"

She explained in very precise terms the bottle is a green bottle with a purple paper in it where the patient is supposed to write instructions about how the medical people should treat him or her if they have an emergency and do not want to be resuscitated.

I asked if this was telescoping an important decision about the recovery process? After all I haven't had a heart attack or a stroke yet or been rushed to hospital in an ambulance choking on my own blood.

Yesterday I was swimming fifty lengths in my local public pool and today I'm being asked when I want to *go under* for the last time. She said she could give me more time to consider the question.

I thanked her and laid back to consider my little green bottle and purple paper and how easy it is for them to float just out of reach over the top.

Chapter 6

The Poisoned Chalice

15th December 2017

The first poisoned chalice in this fight against cancer and chemotherapy contains your taste buds. They are supposed to wither away. I am expecting the worst, but people rarely talk about losing the gift of smell and taste. I set out to investigate.

A friend finished chemotherapy for breast cancer in March 2015 and her taste sensations are not yet back. Cups of coffee, wine and other drinks went from 'diabolic' to slightly metallic and an odd smell that told her something was fundamentally altered in her body.

Another friend (it's surprising how many friends had or have cancer) told me everything did not taste disgusting immediately but a few days later she found her food acrid and acid with a burning taste. She went to an acupuncturist who told her, "'The poison is affecting your liver and over-loading it with heat."

Her antidote was to suck on frozen pineapple pieces and other tangy, lemony citrus kind of flavours to help purify the liver.

Although she hated coffee, tea and chocolate, she didn't lose her appetite completely but also she didn't fancy eating anything and her weight dropped to seven stone.

Her sense of smell was affected. There was no let-up. It wouldn't go away and the build-up was cumulative. Only some years later are her taste buds slowly back on the mend.

I came to the cancer dinner table forewarned, but I was determined not to let my taste buds die. Now maybe this is just luck or a case of mind-over-matter, but after five weeks of chemotherapy wine tastes even better and I'm still addicted to chocolate. This is a small victory and I don't know where the energy comes from to fight it.

Maybe it's in the sea of letters, cards and good wishes that keep my head above water – some from long-time friends, others from strangers, like these.

"I don't really know where to start, but although we have never met I feel that if I don't exactly *know* you then I do know the *man with the shark* and the *voice on the radio*.

"There are some very special people out there who have inspired ideas, notions and theories, and not so many years ago cancer was a dark elephant in the room, not so now, I sincerely live in the hope that one of these clever guys finds a key which unlocks the door for you and those around you.

'You take care, embrace every day and please, please, please once more, get your way, and prove the rest of them wrong. **The man with the shark** *just took back a slice of life and proved the establishment wrong.* I think that you make a good headline, one perhaps only you could write."

Here is a familiar voice that always brings a smile and fills up my *determination tank* –

Dearest Bill

It's only the good who die young and you're nowhere near good enough!

I am indeed shocked to read of your news but drugs and science are improving all the time and there have to be good odds that you'll be able to beat the bastard.

You've never been afraid to prove the Establishment wrong and if the establishment says you have a life expectancy of 18 months then 18 years it must be.

Good luck my friend. You've done so much for Oxfordshire, I hope and pray that Oxfordshire's very fine medical teams can pay the debt the county owes you.

You're the best. All luck, wishes, prayers and love,

Attaboy!

Jane Cranston, High Sheriff of Oxfordshire, 2017/18

Chapter 7

Bucket Lists

22nd December 2017

While children make *wish lists* for Christmas, I'm making a *bucket list* of things to do before I die.

Like children I've often thought about what to include, but now that the time is here, I've hit the empty bucket syndrome because there's a hole in my bucket. "Then fix it, dear Bill," I can hear you say, but I've left it too late.

If you've always wanted to travel – the Seychelles, Machu Picchu, the Pyramids or the Great Barrier Reef -- do it now! Don't wait till you've got cancer because then the travel insurance will be sky high for most destinations and your consultant team will veto many of the other places you want to visit on medical grounds.

Effectively you're grounded with cancer unless you stand up to the system like a friend fighting her second cancer battle. She needed a break from chemotherapy and decided to visit Amsterdam without insurance. She knew it was not one of those calm, quiet destinations but she needed to get away. Her doctors played ball. They topped her up with a blood transfusion and gave her a mini-pharmacy to see her through two days and sent her off. So while not impossible, a plane ticket in your bucket list is a difficult *ask*.

I've always wanted to have a meal at Raymond Blanc's famous restaurant, Le Manoir aux Quat' Saisons, especially since I interviewed him one afternoon and he ordered some coffee for us. The first cup was delivered to our table in the drawing room, the second to our table on the lawn, another was served in the kitchen and a fourth in the garden. Each time M. Blanc clicked his fingers, ordered fresh coffee and then moved on before either of us had a sip of any of these four cups.

It was a case of *The Marx Brothers at Le Manoir* – totally bonkers. But I would like a meal there except now with the cancer I can't eat a full meal. Fortunately I was able to swallow a bowl of onion soup at the opening night of Raymond Blanc's new venture at The Black Horse in Thame --simply succulent.

During my student days I would queue for hours at Covent Garden to buy standing room tickets for one shilling and nine pence to watch Margot Fontaine and Rudolph Nureyev dance. When I was hurdled with the rest of them at the very back of the Royal Opera House I would peep out from behind one of those great carved columns and look up at the best seats in the House – gilded boxes each with a private dining room.

Now a ticket to a box seat at the ROH would be a good addition to any *bucket list*, but a few days ago out of the blue I received an invitation to a box seat and dinner for a production of *The Winters' Tale*. So that's accidently sorted.

Seeds are an important area for any kind of *wish list*. Since I'm always deadheading plants to harvest their seeds, I have a huge collection. I can bag them up and label them for someone else to plant in the summer or I can *take care of business* now. I've planted indoors three hundred seeds of fruit and flowers already, so they can thrive in the new year regardless of whose hand is holding the watering can.

I spent an evening recently with some friends discussing the bucket list question. They were all very helpful and made several suggestions, but I rejected them all. Who needs more adventure, excitement and security when I have it all already... If only I'm prepared to make the effort and look.

When I told my friends I wouldn't change a thing and was perfectly happy with my life as it is, they all smiled and agreed that this was the answer – the best bucket list is to have no bucket list. If you're already feeling fine, you've won this one.

So far in my cancer treatment I've probably been *cooking away* inside with all these drugs pumped into my blood stream. In the new year we should see and hear the *snap, crackle and pop* of the results and find out if anything's working.

Chapter 8

My Zero Immune System

29th December 2017

I have a zero immune system so the smallest scratch or minor cough can turn into blood poisoning or pneumonia. My biggest danger area is a crowd and both Christmas and New Year bring their own crowds

I pole vaulted from an isolation bed in the Churchill Hospital to the middle of holiday crowds in a matter of days, probably because I'm my own worst enemy. It's not that I don't know any better; I've had plenty examples of *good practice*.

A friend with a tumour down her back was not supposed to survive her cancer, but during her treatment she went into self-imposed exile. She avoided crowds by going to out-of-town supermarkets at off-peak hours to avoid people and refused to allow even close friends into her house if they were not in robust health. In particular she wouldn't let any grandparents visit her because their small children tend to collect germs which could be incubating in any unsuspecting, cuddly grandparent.

She even made her family undergo quarantine treatment. When her only son came to visit for lunch while one of his office co-workers had the flu, she forced him to eat lunch with her outside sitting side by side in her garden during February dressed in overcoats, hats, gloves and mouth masks, which must have made eating a bit of a chore.

She disinfected her whole house which was an old stone barn conversion and kept one special chair constantly sprayed with a special solution to protect her against germs. This was her *throne* and nobody else could use it.

Hats off to her, she's still surviving some time later, but that wasn't my way. It's hard to change the habits of a lifetime. As a child I was always the last one out of the sandbox and covered with dirt. Germs must be in the genes because my son, Magnus, at sandbox age managed to crawl onto the kitchen table where we kept the bread and butter and he opened the butter dish and smeared it all over himself, even his hair.

My two daughters took a more militant view. Harriet and Livvy decided to de-germ the house as soon as they heard I was diagnosed with leukaemia. When they found out the consultant advised I should live in a squeaky clean environment they gasped and thought that was an even bigger challenge than the leukaemia.

They put their own lives *on hold* and spent fourteen hours per day for ten days to transform the house. Without warning they took everything at home which included thirty years of collecting precious items, at least *precious* to me, and dumped them in one pile to be sorted out later. So all the Egyptian relics and Peruvian weavings together with boxes of the twenty one pills I have to take each day ended up in what became one huge garbage bin formerly known as our sitting room.

I was shocked and asked them what they were doing. With a straight face Livvy calmly replied, "I'm really going for gold on the mould."

Fine... But when your mental world is turned upside down by a diagnosis of cancer, when all the furniture of your mind which you relied on melts away and then everything in your physical world is turned upside down on a rubbish heap it's a left hook to the jaw and a right punch to the body of your self-image.

The kids said that cleaning the house for me was like looking after a toddler. I didn't have a clue about limiting contact. Even now after months of treatment when a house guest arrived for the New Year celebrations I shook hands and started to talk with him without a second thought that this might be a menace. He had come by London Transport where the only place to sit or stand is where thousands of other people have been doing the same thing. It's probably one of the biggest bug breeding machines in London. Shortly after he arrived we both had to hold out our hands for a spray of the hand sanitizer.

And this is my problem. All the signs are there – *Don't touch! Stand back! Play it safe!* – and despite the warnings, I don't. I hold hands, touch, hug and kiss. I take risks and do all the wrong things. So, on the form where it says *cause of death* finding the answer will be easy.

Chapter 9

Chemotherapy

5th January 2018

My prognosis was a life expectancy of 12 to 18 months and there are now 7 to 13 months remaining.

Celebrating the twelve days of Christmas which end today on the Twelfth Night has been a steep learning curve for me.

If you have cancer and you also have eleven guests, there's nowhere to hide. Everyone lives cheek by jowl and the guests can hear what your jowls are getting up to.

I got sick twenty three times from the chemotherapy. I'm not suggesting twenty three upsets in twelve days is the norm. there is no *normal* because each person responds differently to chemo-therapy and there are vastly different types of *chemo*.

Before you accuse me of being anally retentive in counting the episodes, what else would you do when you are retching your insides out.

I became pretty adept at hiding these explosions. Waitrose has its own free newspaper and I used it to line my basket which at least may protect any tomatoes or avocados I was leaning over. I think the urge to retch may be the excessive stimuli of the red and green colours and the soft shapes, coupled with the muzak stores play. I've heard 'White Christmas' so many times, I'd probably strangle Bing Crosby if he was still around – but what a legacy he left: all that treacle and syrup.

Going to eat at restaurants can be a bit tricky. I always order soup and more soup and then with my mind's eye, I measure the width and depth of the bowl because I may need to use it in an emergency on my way to the toilet. It is surprising how much a soup bowl can hold.

I eat mostly soup because I have no appetite. So the Christmas turkey, ham and salmon didn't tempt me much which is a very positive development because my chemotherapy turned out to be aversion therapy.

I was given my injection treatment at the Day Care Unit for cancer patients at the Churchill Hospital where they plied me daily with tea, coffee and turkey salad sandwiches with mayo on rye. Now I can't even look at a sandwich. I get sick on tea and coffee. Fortunately I wasn't allowed to drink wine, so no problem there. However I can probably manage only one more litre of chocolate fudge brownie ice cream.

I've long since gone off all kinds of pills through the aversion therapy, but the medical profession threatened all kinds of consequences if I don't cooperate. They seem to see me as a suitable case for treatment -- a human equivalent of a goose being fattened up for foie gras.

These pills were not ordinary pills but VIPs and big. One five hundred mg pill got caught in my throat and each swallow turned into a dagger cutting my windpipe.

One of the *blessings* of chemotherapy, at least mine, is that it provides an escape from anything unpleasant through sleep. When the movies or the debates went on for too long I could nod off any time of day.

Of course this *blessing* can't reach the part that a friend of mine with cancer described – At Christmas, when everyone is full of joy and I feel hollowed out, I think: what's the point?

This strange celebration of Christmas tends to reach a peak in our house on New Year's Eve. We light Chinese lanterns and send them into the sky. It's the closest thing to a sacred moment, when we offer something to the air, watch it bounce about tentatively and then take off, flying higher and higher.

It somehow lifts the spirits, but we stand with shoulders hunched and well wishes as this little light goes with the wind. We know it's delicate. We don't know where it's going, but we all hope it won't come crashing down in flames and disaster, although it could. Maybe that's the secret: we know and yet we still go with it. Long may the delicacy be as robust as it is.

Chapter 10

A Day of Rest

12th January 2018

When you have leukaemia and take chemotherapy that knocks out your immune system seven days in a row, you appreciate a day of rest so I was looking forward to a holiday last Sunday.

I had the obligatory double chemo injections mid-morning and promptly threw up. My partner Jane and I were invited to a post New Year's party at noon and there is nothing like champagne to get over chemo and calm down for a leisurely week ahead.

It began slowly with one small drip. I could see the spot of blood on the red tiles. Easy to clean up: not so easy to stop. With no immune system and not much to clot the blood, the nosebleed started at three that afternoon and the drip turned into a tide. It just oozed out.

I ran through three rolls of toilet paper until we rang the hospital at 9.00 pm. By ten I was admitted to the John Radcliffe A & E. What was left of my day of rest went down the drain.

On arrival a piece of paper at the front desk greeted me with suggestions of 16 different boxes I could tick about my nationality. After reading all 16 categories, I was convinced this was a hoax, but it wasn't. The receptionist said she didn't even bother with the question any more.

When she inquired what my problem was I withdrew my hand from my nose for a second and blood coursed all over the place.

We went quickly to triage and down the corridor to the A&E hall. The first Sunday/Monday morning of the New Year was probably typical, but it was definitely hell.

A&E is a large hall with a medical station in the middle and cubicles around two sides. One wall was a large entry portal for the ambulance staff. Interspersed around the room were wheel-chairs and beds full of people who didn't want to be there who were confused and crying out in pain. It was like a theatre where the wounded sat or lay around and watched each other.

I was here because I might bleed to death if I were not treated, but at least I knew why I was there, who was treating me and what to expect. Some of the others didn't and took to the stage in fright.

One woman in a wheel-chair was parked under some spot lights and was holding her arm in a sling.

There are certain English women with prematurely greying hair, a rose complexion and high cheekbones who remain aloof from this kind of drama. Her face was fixed in an *almost* smile with the lips parted, showing her teeth. Behind this façade she was confused and kept asking for the ambulance man to take her home. From time to time her face crumbled, quickly, like lightning -- lips had closed, the chin collapsed and her head sank into a short flood of terms. Then she recovered and renewed her screams for the ambulance man. This was the first act.

The second act was longer. Gracie was desperately seeking Phillip and kept screaming for him in a plaintive way that reached a crescendo when she packed his name 58 times into one minute. She obviously loved Phillip and thought he would save her. At first I was convinced Phillip was her cat, but he later turned out to be her grandson who was at home asleep and expected to visit her at nine in the morning; but she ripped the cold hours of the night with pleas for someone to produce Phillip immediately. He never materialized, but she disappeared after four hours.

The third act began for the captive audience with a man strapped to his bed waiting for an X-ray. He began another soliloquy: "Doctor, nurse! Why leave me like this? Where are you? Take me to my X -ray now." Finally one nurse couldn't take it anymore and politely explained that it was the middle of the night, the X-ray department had a long queue and he would get there as soon as a doctor or nurse was free.

He wasn't happy and demanded immediate treatment. She explained there was no one available, but they could hire a porter to take him. "Would you be prepared to pay for that?" "No!" he screamed and shut up at the break of dawn.

These three acts to the drama featured people who were elderly, frail and confused, but each one could have earned the Golden Globe Award for best tonsils in A&E.

It was heart breaking hell and went on for nine hours and was so riveting no one in the audience was able to look away or block out the sound.

In addition no one in A&E got a minute's sleep that night.

By 8 in the morning with no let-up in the biblical red flood from my nose, I was sent for specialist treatment at the ENT department. The scarf around my neck dragged on the floor as the porter wheeled me out and collected a huge cluster of dirt and dust.

I spent three more hours in ENT after a platelet infusion and an intravenous blood coagulant booster. The doctor released me just in time to travel from the JR to the Churchill Hospital for another round of chemo at 11.00.

When I arrived home at noon after almost 27 hours of my Day of Rest, I noticed a sharp pain in my right arm where the staff had forgot to remove the significantly large and sharp needle of my canula for the blood transfusion.

Then I noticed I was coughing in bed. With a compromised immune system, what next? Pneumonia?

Chapter 11

Bone Marrow Biopsy

19th January 2018

Leukaemia is a liquid cancer that flows through the veins and starts in the bones. And the best way to monitor it is through a bone marrow biopsy.

I was a bone marrow biopsy virgin at the start of treatment and my consultant was determined I should stay that way. "I've booked a biopsy in two hours at one o'clock this afternoon and admitted you to hospital now, so go to bed, relax and I'll see you shortly."

I didn't buy into this: "No, I'm going home first to change my pants. Hasn't your mother told you to make sure you wear clean pants because you never know when you'll end up in hospital? So my mother's penny has dropped. I'll be back by one."

Reluctantly she agreed on the condition that when I got home I would not *Google* bone marrow biopsy. "Some of the pod casts on *You Tube* are misleading."

During the trip home I had a car accident and no time to Google. She was waiting for me in the bone marrow biopsy room wearing a plastic apron covering her clothes and sending out the signals that she wanted to protect her tasteful suit from my blood and gore. I froze, but I wasn't going to show her any fear.

At this stage no one had yet explained exactly what a bone marrow biopsy was and there were no clues in the room, no tools in sight, no drills, no hammers or saws and no anaesthetist. So I was still in the dark.

"If you hop on the bed and lie on your left hand side, I'll just pop in the local." That could have meant she was going for a pint at The Butcher's Arms, but no... It meant a needle in my pelvis to deaden the pain.

She was reassuring: "I give the drug a long time to work so the patient feels little pain." I could hear the clank of metal behind my back. Had I walked into a dungeon or an operating theatre?

Then Nurse Biggles knelt beside me and held my hand. Her job, although she didn't say, was to gauge my pain by how firmly I gripped her hand and communicate silently with her eyes to Frankenstein who was standing out of sight behind my back wielding the knife, chainsaw or drill.

It was a doddle. No pain at all and I shared a few jokes with Biggles. Frankenstein was most efficient at ... What? I still don't know and prefer the bliss of ignorance. But it went very smoothly, so smoothly I swung out of the *theatre* bed and walked back to my room immediately.

Then it hit me! I hadn't had any lunch and I was hungry and besides I deserved a treat.

In the hospital corridor back to my room were these condescending posters showing people with walking sticks and the headline: *Have You Taken Your Walk Yet?*

I ripped one of the posters off the wall and showed the ward nurse and told her I was going for my daily stroll. Then I marched straight out of the Churchill Hospital with a huge needle still protruding from my forearm and still half sedated fifteen minutes after a surgical procedure, I took a one mile round trip walk to the Waitrose Shop in Headington to get some Ben and Jerry's Chocolate Fudge Ice Cream.

I was back within the hour. They thought I was on a leash following their instructions to get some exercise in the hospital world. I knew I was escaping into dessert land.

But my experience, with the bone marrow biopsy, not the ice cream, is nothing to go by, even though I've had a second biopsy which was also pain free.

A few weeks ago after she had held the hand of another patient in a similar procedure, Nurse Biggles was spotted on the wards with her arm in a sling.

The patient's grip on her hand was more than she bargained for. The pain from the bone marrow biopsy prompted the patient to squeeze so hard Biggles needed an X-ray to see if any bones were broken and she wasn't holding any more hands for some time.

I hope she heals in time for my third bone marrow biopsy in a month's time, which should show what is happening in the minefield of my bones where my life's chances are battling it out with the medical prognosis that I'm likely to be dead by the end of this year.

Chapter 12

Medical Language

26th January 2018

Some medical people have a problem with language. They may use it to keep patients in the dark or to gloss over *difficult* (read *life threatening*) situations or even as a power play.

When my cancer trip started in the nurses' office of my GP, I simply asked her to inspect a leg ulcer. She was alarmed and asked for another nurse and a GP to inspect. All three told me if the infection got any worse or if I felt *unwell* I should ring a special direct number she gave me and immediately go to the emergency ward.

I didn't understand what she meant by *unwell* and asked what would happen if I missed the symptoms. She took a long breath, leaned forward in her chair which was significantly higher than mine, stared at me, said nothing and brought out her two index fingers to make the sign of a cross as if warning off a vampire. Maybe she felt uncomfortable about saying Y*ou could die if this infection gets into the blood stream*. That was it -- my first non-verbal communication about my unnamed disease: cancer.

On the hospital wards language was also a problem area. I've had several scans -- CAT, MRI, and *CT Renal and Contrast both*. Of course I have no idea, and they did not explain on paper what these scans meant. I pressed the doctors and they finally said they found some lesions. Where? "Near the pancreas." *What does this mean?* "We're not sure." I eventually got out of them that this could be the start of pancreatic cancer.

On another admission to hospital I was given a spacious room all to myself. It was luxurious with my own shower and a terrific view. I stayed there five days without knowing I was in an isolation room.

The medics had located *something akin* to MRSA, the drug-resistant bug that many hospitals have and that can kill you. Fortunately my particular bug was slightly different than MRSA and called MSSA. The first *S* means it is *susceptible* to treatment.

I had no idea I was going through such a close shave with death, but all the staff, including *visitors, porters and domestics* knew because there was a big sign outside my door that read -- *Enhanced Contact Precautions (source isolation)* that told staff to *decontaminate hands, wear gloves and aprons and/or long sleeve gowns on entering the room. Discard after use and decontaminate your hands.*

There I was, inside my decontaminated cage, happy as Larry without any clue that visitors must *report to the Nurse-in-Charge or seek advice from the nursing staff before entering this room.*

When I was discharged I happened to see this notice outside my room and ripped it off the wall as a souvenir... Of what? Openness, inclusion and respect for the patient or control and the view that it is better to keep the patient in the dark?

I'm out of the hospital for now, but I don't know how long that will last, and I don't know how my cancer treatment is working, if at all. I got a letter this week saying the appointment with my consultant has been cancelled and rescheduled five weeks later to 1st March.

In the meantime I'm enjoying my freedom, doing the small, daily things in life, like going shopping at Tesco's in Summertown. The cancer helps you see things differently, like the guy who sits in front of Tesco's not quite begging but he's right there at the door when you leave, sitting on what must be a pretty hard and cold piece of the footpath. He's unusual because he has one trouser leg pulled up to the knee to expose a large, angry-looking, bright red scab of an ulcer on his shin.

I've passed him on several trips, but this time I stopped because he caught my eye and motioned for me to come over. It was the first time I had really looked at him. He returned my gaze straight on and said "How's the treatment going? I've been reading your columns in the Oxford Mail and I hope it's working."

He stopped me in my tracks with his directness. There was no agenda. He wasn't looking for a handout and I didn't give him anything. He just wanted to engage. So we talked. Then after a while he said, "You know, you have the ability to touch people. You've got a bit of God in you and you don't even know it," and we parted company. But if I had to give a quarter time score on the way people use words, it would be science – zero, beggars – one.

Chapter 13

The Blood Cancer Triage Unit

2nd February 2018

The blood cancer triage unit at the Churchill Hospital is designed to enable immediate treatment and instant access to hospital care and drugs for those very ill patients in danger of death. I've used it three times and I know how valuable it can be. It's a life saver... Until it isn't.

Last week on Monday I nicked my chin while shaving, just a scratch you wouldn't even notice, the size of a piece of dry oatmeal mix before you boil it up for breakfast.

My leukaemia and chemotherapy combined have wiped out my immune system so something as innocent as a shaving *nick* can open the floodgates to bacteria into my blood system, bacteria that can be far from innocent.

Not surprisingly, my chin became infected and the red halo surrounding the cut grew into the size of a ten pence piece while I tried to contain it with antiseptic dressings. All this effort proved to be of no avail; by Wednesday it had grown into the size of a fifty pence piece.

I didn't want to bother the medics unnecessarily so I kept my head down and kept my chin as protected as possible; but this infection was on the march and now covered most of my chin.

By Thursday I realized this was not only serious but was not going away. During the night I woke up with a difficulty swallowing, but I still refused to call the triage department at such an antisocial hour as 4.00 in the morning.

When I woke up at 9.00 on Friday, I could see the infection had spread from something on the surface of my chin to a painful inflammation of areas inside my neck and head -- my throat and mouth. My whole jaw was so painful and swollen and frozen in a way that made my jaw protrude and give me a Dan Dare look. The alarm bells rang when I discovered I couldn't talk and the pain was invading my cheeks. However I kept taking my temperature and I hadn't reached the cut-off point of 37.5 degrees which is taken as the official gauge to say *someone has a temperature*.

I knew that if the infection got into my blood stream and I got blood poisoning or sepsis this could prove fatal in a very short time. When your body turns against you it can do that very quickly.

My partner called the blood cancer triage department *hot line* which we were given three times because the line was busy. When she got through she explained the infection was starting to interfere with my throat, swallowing and breathing.

The main question the triage person had was whether or not I had a temperature. When she replied that I didn't, they cut the conversation short, said their service was not the appropriate one and told me to go see my GP.

So we rang the GP's office and the duty doctor made an appointment within forty minutes. The GP took a very short time, probably a matter of minutes, to refer me to the triage unit. He wrote a covering note and rang the unit several times to alert them of my arrival and got no answer. Because he was having trouble getting through, he finally told me to get myself to the hospital and he would continue trying to reach them while I was on my way.

When I arrived to deliver the GP's letter, I found three medics on reception and one told me "I have no idea why you are here. We have not been informed of your arrival.' And he just stood there for a moment looking at me. My thought was: "Oh that's that then. Maybe I should just go away." But I knew this was too serious; so I stood my ground.

After reading the letter they took me into the triage care unit which had four beds and two patients. They were not obviously swept off their feet with emergency admissions at first sight, but perhaps I couldn't see the whole picture that the three people on reception knew about.

Once beyond this door and inside the unit the care was faultless, the nurses efficient, helpful, good natured and humorous. They gave me an immediate injection of antibiotics even before taking and testing my blood.

Soon a porter came to wheel me to a room where I received treatment for three days. Once again the thoroughness and attention to details of the doctors and nurses was excellent.

I can talk and swallow now and the infection has gone back to the size of a fifty pence piece and I no longer had a chin that looks like Dan Dare.

I choose to hold the blood cancer triage unit with respect and esteem in spite of the treatment I received at the point of entry and the very real difficulties I experienced in trying to get through the door.

I understand there have to be guard dogs at the gate, but some of these are obviously more *people friendly* than others. But since I may have to use this service in the future, I'll try to keep you posted on these pooches.

Chapter 14

Is My Treatment Working?

9th February 2018

Six of the months of my life expectancy have passed and I'm half way to one third through treatment depending on how it works out. So the big question at this point is how is the treatment working?

I'm still on the experimental cancer drug trial taking something that could be a break-through drug that could offer hope for millions of patients or it may fail or I may not respond to this particular treatment which could work for others.

It's a slippery and rocky road but after six months I should be able to get some bearings of where I am on this trip. This last week was a time of reckoning. Is the drug showing signs of working or not?

Alarm bells started to ring when my last treatment cycle was put on hold and I had an unscheduled bone marrow biopsy which gives an up-to-date reading of the progression of the leukaemia.

We've been getting indications of the state of play through my blood tests. The nurses take my blood samples two or three times a week and get between ten and twenty vials of blood which are sent off to the trial administration in Switzerland and the United States and of course here to the Churchill Hospital.

A special meeting was scheduled with my consultant after the biopsy and extra blood samples. The questions are –

can we tell what's happening to the disease and if the treatment is not working, then what?

I arrived for the appointment on time and the nurse weighed me and said I had not lost any weight in the six months of treatment. Apparently that's encouraging. Then came the moment that mattered, the results of my blood composition straight from the bone marrow biopsy where the cancer cells are counted in a sample one-by-one by hand.

When I started treatment these cancer cells measured 38% of the blood. The target of the treatment was to cut them back to 5% or below but maybe as high as 10%. The consultant revealed that the cancer cells had not dropped but had risen from 38% at the start to 56% now. The percentages were going in the wrong direction.

This came as a shock because I believed I was onto a winner with this new experimental treatment and I was expecting to see a reduction in the cancer cells. The consultant confirmed that by this stage in the treatment cycles for most of the participants in this world-wide trial, 70% of them showed reductions and the expectation was that the cancer cells would now be in the 5% to 10% region.

I've never felt like I was drowning before. I used to be a lifeguard. I've saved a fair few people and I've seen the look on their faces when they were not waving but drowning. This was a situation where I was not waving.

A quiet panic kicks in, if there is such a thing, and the questions you've fought off at the back of your brain march to the front in an unruly crowd: *Is this it – the end of the road?* Was my one best hope of the break-through drug a vain, empty one? Where do we go from here? I felt like I had let myself down. Why wasn't I on the winning side?

The consultant had the final say to stop the trial or not. He told me I looked very healthy and asked me how I felt, but he put the question in a curious way that caught me off-balance. "Do you sometimes feel like a cancer fraud, like you don't really have the disease and shouldn't be here?" When I nodded, he asked what percentage of the time did I feel that way. I had to think about that one and replied that yes, I did feel like a fraud about 80% of the time.

His reply was straightforward. "Good, because in spite of the numbers, something is happening in your bone marrow and blood. The red cells count is steady and rising and your platelet counts have risen from 8 to 45 which is increasing your ability to fight infection. If something weren't going on you would have been in and out of the hospital like a yo-yo.

"We still have three more cycles of treatment to go through and some patients don't show any cancer cell reduction until the later stages. Yes, 70% respond in the first six cycles but 90% respond by 9 cycles, We can't tell what's working, but something is changing. So let's continue with the trial."

Chapter 15

My Family – Public Enemy Number One

16th February 2018

Both the cancer and the chemotherapy shoot holes through the immune system. Many cancer patients practically have no immunity to the diseases and bugs that live all around us and on our skins.

The public is not enemy number one; it turns out my family is!

Jane, my partner, has come down with this year's version of the Aussie H3N2 flu. She's been in bed for four weeks and says she is now coming down with a re-infection. She coughs like a trooper and either clears her throat or goes into a coughing fit once every minute. (I counted).

She's dizzy, usually has a headache and stays in bed. And she's given it to our son who has been ill with the symptoms for the last two weeks. He ran a temperature of 40.1. When my temperature hits 37.5 degrees the medics examine me in hospital.

So how am I coping with this double dose of flu under my nose? For some reason I have escaped that particular problem and yet I'm living with it night and day and I'm supposed to be the one with the compromised immune system? I'm probably tempting fate by raising the matter.

The headlines make for cautionary reading: "Brits have been urged to dose themselves with vitamin C as the country faces the worst Aussie flu epidemic in 50 years. Almost 100,000 Australians have fallen ill to H3N2, their most severe outbreak on record."

I must have an unusual immune system if it keeps protecting me when all those around are dropping like flies. Of course I am taking one anti-fungal and three anti-viral tablets each day, so that may be part of the answer to this mystery.

But perhaps I should start on vitamin C. Alternative medical approaches to treating cancer have been cropping up since I started writing these articles. I've already read a book on apricot kernels, but my experience with vitamin C is closer to home.

A friend was lecturing in the States at MIT in the 1970s and worked with Linus Pauling, one of only four people to have won two unshared Nobel prizes -- Chemistry in 1954 and Peace in 1962. My friend was diagnosed with his second bout of cancer and given just four months to live. Linus Pauling got very interested in this and told my friend that most animals make their own vitamin C in large amounts. In humans, the gene for this ability has mutated and no longer works properly. Linus advised my friend to take 15 grams of vitamin C with 15 grams of sodium ascorbate and mix this with V8 vegetable juice and take the mixture every day. He does and is still alive and kicking at 80.

Then there is frankincense which researchers at the University of Leicester argue can diminish and remove cancer spreads or metastases.

Leukaemia is a blood cancer and does not have solid metastases, but simply goes all around the body already as a liquid cancer. In some cases, like mine, leukaemia does migrate to the skin and I have leukaemia sores. Frankincense oil can be taken internally or used externally. Perhaps it would help to use it on my sores? Or is this just a myth of Biblical proportions?

Chapter 16

Victim, Sufferer, an Embarrassment

23 February 2018

When you get cancer you become another person, maybe several – *victim, sufferer, an embarrassment*. Perhaps this is based on fear – they don't want to know about the disease that is more likely than not to be the one which will lay them low, or they might not want to be part of the long goodbye that ends in death.

Most people make a genuine effort to reach out. The problem is most of them don't know what to say or do, but then, neither does the person with cancer.

Do I hate my body, in particular my blood because that's the very thing that is killing me? No, that way is a lose-lose situation. I've decided to embrace the cancer, but at the same time to fight it head-on like you would do in a boxing match with an opponent you respect.

I remember my GP Ann McPherson before she died a few years ago with pancreatic cancer saying, "Sometimes life just deals you a very shitty hand."

The cancer victim or sufferer stereotype has pretty much died the death. I have: "Can we still count on you? I don't come across too many who are angry on my behalf or simply befuddled and bemused.

Most people who want to treat the cancer person as *invisible* have disappeared. Now almost everyone wants to engage, especially those in the medical profession. But if I come across anyone else with big round Bambi eyes who reaches out to put a slightly moist hand on my arm and shoulder and asks softly, *But how are you, Bill?* I will go join a gym so I can let them know how many pounds I am bench pressing this week and compare it to last week, so they can answer their own question.

The old question *are you a player or are you a watcher* is well in evidence. People want to know if you are one of the actors ready to take to the stage and engage or if you've decided to be part of the audience and watch from now on. The questions are leading and not so subtle: "Can we still count on you? Remember when? Would you still be up for that? I don't want to add any pressure, but could you please?"

I can understand why so many cancer people prefer to keep quiet about their disease, keep their heads down and withdraw or almost disappear, because they have to go over the same ground again and again each time they meet someone and it's very private terrain.

I've chosen to go public precisely to flag up questions like these so people can see there's not much of a way forward or back. You just have to play your hand as best you can with skill, hope and a Mona Lisa smile.

You can even become the pet project of some members of the public. Currently I've been taken under the wing of a rough sleeper who spends his days on the streets of Summertown. One very cold, and from his look, not very successful day, he took me aside this week and said, "You've got to beat this. One night go home and say to yourself – I can win – the next night say I'm going to win – and on the third – I will win."

The next night he shouted at me from across the street as I was getting into my car "Remember AMP – attitude makes you positive." And this from a man who has spent the day *not quite begging*, on the streets of Oxford.

I do get the *heroic* response when people tell me how brave I'm being. This one is not too difficult. I tell people I've been telling stories most of my life over the airwaves, in print and on TV, and I don't know how to stop and can't help it.

Generally I don't get the verbal treatment, more the physical with lots of hugs. At one dinner party I thought the cook was going to throw me into the pot when she grabbed me around the neck, drilled into my eyes with hers and repeated over and over – "You're going to beat this, you've just got to."

One response was very simple: "Well, there's really nothing to say, is there?" And my friend and I raised a glass of wine to life.

Chapter 17

Preparing to Die – or Live?

2nd MARCH, 18

I'm still on a world-wide trial of a new drug to treat the problem. I'm not responding, but even now, seven months later I feel fine. So we're continuing the treatment. The question now though is how should we treat the balance I find myself caught in: should I start preparing to die or to live?

It's March, the sun and the garden are beckoning. It reminds me of the day I spent with Michael and Anne Heseltine in their arboretum in Thenford near Banbury. At the end of the day I wanted to go beyond gardening, so I suggested to Michael there is a particular view that if you live in the country on a farm and go through the seasons -- birth, growth, withering, death and rebirth – there's almost a spiritual aspect of all that. I asked if there was a spiritual aspect to his garden.

His answer left a question mark over the conversation. "I wouldn't call it a spiritual aspect, but very much an awareness of the rotational aspect of nature itself. To me, one of the formative moments which always comes, and it's always memorable, is that day when you are wandering around in March, probably slightly stooped, probably looking down, and suddenly you feel the warmth of the sun on your back and it straightens you up. I'm now very conscious it happens about the same time every year. Now you can say, well fine, what's that mean? What it means of course is that's exactly what every bulb, every tree, every plant feels as well when the natural cycle of spring comes back."

So I have to make some decisions. I've already planted inside about three hundred seedlings. Most are up and going great guns. When I started this project I didn't know who would finish it. Now maybe it looks like I could. I'm caught in that balance. Do I clear the rubbish in the garden from last year, get out the pitchfork and start to design my horticultural dream or do I let the garden go to seed and weed?

My USA University class reunion is coming up the first weekend of June. It's a big one, the fiftieth. Georgetown University and Washington DC look beautiful in the springtime and I'm sure most of the classmates will be there including Bill Clinton.

I'd like to go, but in June will I still be up for the travel and feel like a party?

Then there is the audio book of *The Hunting of the Shark* that sculptor John Buckley and I put up in my new Headington House back in 1986. I've long wanted to turn that saga into more of a book portrait rather than simply an audio book, especially since many of the major players are still alive and could play themselves in the drama, including Lord Heseltine who gave the Shark planning permission when he was Secretary of State for the Environment in the early 1990s. The next birthday of the Shark is 9 August, so I've got to start planning that now if it's ever going to happen.

I've long wanted to write a book about the Baby Boomer Generation to distinguish our dreams and aspirations from those of the *X* generation or that of the Millennials. We pushed the boundaries in ways they didn't even think about... Like hitching a lift on a US Air Force plane at the height of the Viet Nam War and shortly after the assassination of a president from Andrew's Air Force base where the President's plane, Air Force One, is kept. I had my first sauna fifty years ago in a sweat lodge with five braves and a medicine man after riding a donkey down a side canyon of the Grand Canyon to spend a week with the Havasupai native Americans on their reservation with no electricity. If it exists now, it will have electricity and it won't have a *sweat lodge* due to health and safety regulations.

I am probably the only person ever to head butt a rather awkward and out-of-sorts guest after the funeral mass of President John Kennedy at St Matthew's Cathedral courtyard called Richard Nixon.

And I sailed a felucca, a centuries old sailing boat made from a hollowed out tree, down a crocodile infested Nile at night while my *guide* was having an appendix attack flat on the floor and my son was tied to the mast to stop him from being tipped overboard during a storm.

It was going to be called *Things I can't Do Anymore When I'm 64*. I'm now 73 and the question is -- will I ever complete it? If I don't start these things I'll have no way of knowing whether or not they could ever exist.

Yes, I have a few choices to make and not much guidance.

Chapter 18

Ignorance, Faith and Hope

9th March 2018

Not many people write about the experience of getting chemotherapy. There's a reason for that. All chemotherapies and their host users are different, yet all chemos are the same – they are poison of course because their purpose is to kill the cancer cells.

Most chemotherapy is not targeted only on the cancer cells, but hits all cells in your body. My chemo, azacitadene, has not changed and there has been no significant development of it since it was introduced into this county thirty odd years ago so at this stage it is a very old and crude tool.

What has changed in those years is the discovery of new drugs to deal with the side effects on administration, those *masks* that hide the harm, nausea, sickness and danger while you are taking them.

I haven't found the right combination yet – the drug that lets you take the chemo and camouflages the bad bits. This isn't too serious because my routine is to take chemo for seven straight days in a row along with a new experimental trial drug and then take nothing but a holiday for three weeks. So after one month we repeat the cycle. I'm on cycle seven and this is my chemo week which I've taken with three different masking drugs and once without any. So I can tell you what's really going on, at least for me. It's a very dark and disturbing place and you don't ever want to go there.

This is the story they don't tell you.

It starts with ignorance, faith and hope. It has to... Otherwise why would anyone willingly agree to be seriously poisoned, go into a small cubicle, raise their shirt and offer up their stomachs for two injections, one on either side? You can look away and tell yourself it's not happening, but there are tell-tale signs at the end of a week. The nurse is struggling to find areas for the injections that are not inflamed and your whole stomach area is swollen, lumpy and feels like some thug has been beating you up with a baseball bat swinging at full force.

That's how you start out, but why do you keep going? It's not ignorance anymore because you know *the drill*. Faith and hope are all that's left. You've got to believe very strongly that taking this poison would do anyone more good than harm. And you've got to hope that this particular chemo combo out of all the ones available is the right one for you. Without those twin pillars of personal power, no one would go through with this.

Of course there are the *mask pills* that can be taken to disguise the poison. My first pill, which was supposed to stop the nausea and vomit, actually induced those very symptoms before I even had the chemo. The second one had side effects I wasn't prepared to tolerate and the third simply extended the period of nausea.

Those are the reasons why I tried taking the chemo without the masks. I've been on a small yacht in the middle of the Atlantic during a gale and tied myself to the mast so I could experience the full force of nature. I'd rather repeat that then repeat the experience of the full force of the chemo.

In films, directors often try to portray satanic possession by using vomit. Remember that scene in *The Exorcist* of the girl Regan lying on her back in bed and projecting a violent stream of vomit straight into the air three or four feet high?

That can't happen with me because I know it's a mistake to eat anything around the time the nurses inject the chemo. It's better to take the poison on an empty stomach. But only slightly better because then you get the *dry heaves*. The sensation is like somebody putting their hand down your throat, trying to get a grip of any part of your stomach to rip out, over and over. In my case it lasted for two hours.

This is a very bleak, physical time and a dangerous mental area.

Chapter 19

Odious Comparisons

18th March 2018

I've known the columnist George Monbiot for over thirty years, and I have a lot of respect for George. On Wednesday this week he wrote in *The Guardian*, "I have been diagnosed with prostate cancer, but I'm happy."

How does he shake *happiness* out of those bones? He reaches for comparisons. How does his cancer compare to the situation his friends find themselves in with other medical or family conditions? How does it compare with what might have been a worse case? How does it fall in comparison with other possible Monbiot disasters? And he concludes that the old Dickensian approach *Cheer Up It could be worse* is much better than the current vogue of *Look* or *Hello!* magazines prompting us to imagine how much better things could be.

When you've got cancer all comparisons are odious. All cancers and their treatments are individual. Instead of seeing ourselves as deprived of what others possess -- good health -- which as Monbiot points out is a formula for misery, he uses it as a way to count his blessings.

I like the direction of travel, but how far do you get if you go down that road? Isn't the point of a tumour to change it if you can, but above all to understand, to be *of the moment*, not to compare but to be part of the here and now. Maybe that's what George was getting at.

But I do make more than my fair share of comparisons each time I walk into the Day Treatment Unit at the Churchill

Hospital. The is where hundreds, maybe thousands, of cancer patients get treated each week.

They check in usually with a friend or family member, often in a wheelchair or with mobility chairs, but when they do walk, they usually walk behind and slower than their partner. But make no mistake, there is a determination, a steeliness in the person with cancer that says loud and clear *I know what's going on. I know where I'm going and I'm going to beat this.*

These people are just the ordinary Joe and Josephine from across Oxfordshire, Buckinghamshire and Northamptonshire and beyond, but when you walk into that group you can feel the energy and the power, and see it in their eyes and the way they move.

Some may have good days; others may have bad days, but I suspect not one of us is thinking of that. We're not even thinking about all those other numberless disasters that could have laid us low or imagining how much better things could be.

In our mind's eyes we don't see the rich lists and the power lists filling our newspapers or the reality stars that have stepped from behind the television screen into our imaginations.

We are unaware of the billions of pounds spent on marketing and advertising to *create an infrastructure of comparison that ensure we see ourselves as deprived of what others possess.*

Nope, we're just thinking of moving one foot in front of the other. Maybe we are two feet behind our 'minders' or loved ones, but we're walking. We'll get to where we have to go for now. Then we'll make a new plan and go somewhere different. But we're on the move, and it's a privilege to be part of it.

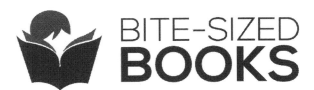

Bite-Sized Lifestyle Books are designed to provide insights and ideas about our lives and the pressures on all of us and what we can do to change our environment and ourselves.

They are deliberately short, easy to read, books helping readers to gain a different perspectives. They are firmly based on personal experience and where possible successful actions and aren't academic or research-based. They are written with hope and optimism.

The most successful people all share an ability to focus on what really matters, keeping things simple and understandable. As Stephen Covey famously said, "The main thing is to keep the main thing, the main thing".

But what exactly is the main thing?

Bite-Sized books were conceived to help answer precisely that question crisply and fast and, of course, be engaging to read, written by people who are experienced and successful in their field.

The brief? Distil the "main things" into a book that can be read by an intelligent non-expert comfortably in around 60 minutes. Make sure the book enables the reader with specific ideas and plenty of examples drawn from real life. In some cases the books are a virtual mentor.

Bite-Sized Books don't cover every eventuality, but they are written from the heart by successful people who are happy to share their experience with you and give you the benefit of their success.

We have avoided jargon – or explained it where we have used it as a shorthand – and made few assumptions about the reader, except that they are literate and numerate, and that they can adapt and use what we suggest to suit their own, individual purposes.

They can be read straight through at one easy sitting and then used as a support while you are thinking further about the issues that most of us face.

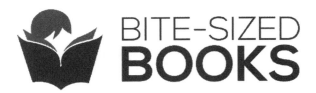

Bite-Sized Books Catalogue

Business Books

Ian Benn
>Write to Win
>>How to Produce Winning Proposals and
RFP Responses

Matthew T Brown
>Understand Your Organisation
>>An Introduction to Enterprise Architecture
Modelling

David Cotton
>Rethinking Leadership
>>Collaborative Leadership for Millennials
and Beyond

Richard Cribb
>IT Outsourcing: 11 Short Steps to Success
>>An Insider's View

Phil Davies
>How to Survive and Thrive as a Project Manager
>>The Guide for Successful Project
Managers

Paul Davies
>Developing a Business Case
>>Making a Persuasive Argument out of
Your Numbers

Don Sharp
>Nothing Happens Until You Sell Something
>>A Personal View of Selling Techniques

Christopher Hosford
>Great Business Meetings! Greater Business Results
>>Transforming Boring Time-Wasters into Dynamic Productivity Engines

Lifestyle Books

Anna Corthout
>Alive Again
>>My Journey to Recovery

Phil Davies
>Don't Worry Be Happy
>>A Personal Journey

Phil Davies
>Feel the Fear and Pack Anyway
>>Around the World in 284 Days

Regina Kerschbaumer
>Yoga Coffee and a Glass of Wine
>>A Yoga Journey

Gillian Perry
>Capturing the Celestial Lights
>>A Practical Guide to Imagining the Northern Lights

Arthur Worrell
>A Grandfather's Story
>>Arthur Worrell's War

Public Affairs Books

Eben Black
> Lies Lunch and Lobbying
>> PR, Public Affairs and Political
>> Engagement – A Guide

John Mair and Richard Lance Keeble – Editors
> Investigative Journalism Today
>> Speaking Truth to Power

Christian Wolmar
> Wolmar for London
>> Creating a Grassroots Campaign in a
>> Digital Age